Homeb
Square Dancing, Creekside
Conversations, & Living Together

A Daughter's Journey Through
the Sandwich Generation

Sally Kauffman

Sally Kauffman
Connect with Sally:
SallyKauffman1953@gmail.com

Ordering Information:
Quantity sales. Special discounts are available on quantity purchases by corporations, associations, and others. For details, contact Sally at SallyKauffman1953@gmail.com

Homebound Harmony: Square Dancing, Creekside Conversations, & Living Together A Daughter's Journey Through the Sandwich Generation
Sally Kauffman. — 1st ed.

ISBN: 979-8-3302272-9-7
ISBN E-Book: 979-8-3302273-0-3

PRINTED IN THE UNITED STATES OF AMERICA.

In memory of my parents. You lived with me in the last years of your lives. Thank you for being with me, teaching me, and loving me. You showed me strength, kindness, and how to keep going, no matter what.

I dedicate this book to you both. Your love and support mean everything to me. You've made me who I am, and I'll always be grateful.

TABLE OF CONTENTS

Loving my parents in their last years along with suggestions if you should find yourself in the same situation

This is not a book on advice, just my story and suggestions on what I learned in the course of being a part of the sandwich generation.

So, what is the sandwich generation? I looked up many definitions and they all go along with; The sandwich generation is a generation of people who care for their aging parents while supporting their own children, may feel overwhelmed and stretched thin as they try to balance the demands of multiple generations and may feel "sandwiched" between the needs of two generations, often leading to feelings of stress and financial strain.

This, I found, can be particularly challenging for those who are also working full-time and trying to balance the demands of their job with the responsibilities of caregiving. I just found a Club Sandwich definition which probably fits me a little better.

As defined by Carol Abaya, a journalist, those in their 50s-60s sandwiched between aging parents, adult children and grandchildren, or those in their 30s-40s, with young children, aging parents and grandparents.

The Beginning

I always wanted to learn some kind of dance. You know when you're a kid, and you dream of being all dressed up, dancing, having fun, and being the absolute best? That's what I thought of when I dreamed of taking a dance class.

So, in March 2006, I signed up for a belly dancing class.

Many years before that, I had visited one of my daughters when she lived in Georgetown. I never drove there because the roads were always one-way, and I could never figure them out. Instead, I would take the local train into Philadelphia and then Amtrak to Washington, DC. From there, I would hop onto the Metro and walk to her house. I always enjoyed walking, seeing the people, and browsing the shops. One shop had these belly dance outfits. I must have stopped in there every time I passed by and browsed through all the outfits. Eventually, I went all in and bought the complete outfit. I mean everything: the skirt, belt, bra, scarf, hip scarf, headband, earrings, finger cymbals, and a ring for my hand. I took it home, put it in my closet, and there it stayed.

Back to the class I signed up for. I was so excited. I remember getting to the class and deciding what to do with my cell phone. Mind you, I hardly ever used it but had to make a decision. I left the phone in my car and went in. I really enjoyed the class. Though I didn't learn any moves in the first class, I thought I could have fun.

After the class, I was so excited to return the next week, which was unusual for me. I walked to the car with a new sense of excitement and adventure. When I got in the car, I grabbed my phone and noticed all the buttons were flashing.

I had seven messages. A few were from my oldest daughter and several from my father. My heart raced as I listened to the messages. My father was crying and said, "Can you come quickly? I don't know what's happening." He was very scared.

You see, my mother and father never wanted to go to a doctor. They each had their own doctor but went very rarely, usually just for their annual physicals. My mother, in the past, made appointments just to get her prescriptions filled. My father was only on one prescription, and they both believed that good food was their path to good health.

Apparently, my 81-year-old mother had not been feeling well that morning and had stayed in bed later than usual. My father was bringing her meals upstairs. After resting all day and eating her dinner, she thought she was feeling better. They were supposed to go square dancing that evening. She got up from her bed and decided she wanted to jump on her rebounder (a mini trampoline). She liked to rebound every day, and today was no exception. She wanted to bounce. But this time, she collapsed next to the rebounder.

My father heard a loud thump and went running upstairs. He called me but couldn't reach me, so he called my oldest daughter, who then called me too.

My excitement from class quickly turned into an unexpected catastrophe. I called my daughter and let her know I was on my way to the hospital.

When I arrived at the hospital, I found my father, who was very upset and distraught. "What do I do?" he asked.

I did my best to comfort him and calm his mind. We needed to wait for the doctors to let us know what was going on with my mother, his wife.

Eventually, the doctor came into the room to let us know she had a stroke. It was a right-sided hemisphere stroke, which left her left side weak, made her aphasic (unable to speak), and caused difficulty swallowing.

Earlier that day was the last time he heard her voice. She would no longer be able to express her thoughts – and we knew my mother always had lots to share. This would be one of the most challenging things for my father to deal with from her stroke.

Returning to square dancing, my parents had been square dancing and round dancing for many years, at least thirty years. They had dances at different venues at least two to three times a week. They used to go to many square dance conventions around the United States. They were due to go to a dance that evening. They never made it to that one, and as my father said, they never went square dancing again. They had asked me if I wanted to square dance in the past, but I always said no, not interested.

A New Beginning

Mom was in the hospital for about two weeks, and my father was told she would need a rehabilitation center. Every day, my 89-year-old father drove to the hospital to spend the day by her side. He stayed with her, doing what he could to keep her company. In the evening, he would go home, watch some baseball—he loved the Phillies—and then go to sleep, only to do it all again the next day.

When she was transferred to the rehabilitation center, he maintained the same routine, though the drive was much longer. As the days and weeks went by, she recuperated little by little. She grew stronger but still struggled to swallow her food without choking. The rehab team was wonderful to both her and my father. They reassured him that they were doing everything they could, and he could see her getting stronger day by day.

Unfortunately, the decision was made to insert a feeding tube in her stomach. My father learned how to operate the feeding tube, hang the formula, and clear the tube after feeding. He managed all her care. Having been a mechanic and later working in an office supply store, he knew how to fix things. He liked to build things with wood, creating cabinets, shelving, and a coffee table in their house. Naturally, he picked up handling the tube feeding and caring for my mother with no problem at all.

You have to understand my father—he did not like to bother anyone. He wouldn't think of asking me to stay home from work to help care for Mom, so I went to work every day and visited them every afternoon after work.

After several weeks of Mom being in rehab, my father called me one day to tell me the social worker wanted to have a meeting with him. He knew Mom was getting stronger, and he had a strong feeling they wanted to place her in a nursing home. This worried him greatly. Not to mention, two of their six grandchildren were coming to visit to see their grandmother and grandfather. He asked if I would come with him to the meeting, and of course, I said yes. Naturally, Dad made the appointment as late as possible in the afternoon so I wouldn't have to miss work.

Here's a little backstory for you.

My parents had lived in a split-level home for the last fifty-three years, and Dad knew Mom would not be able to maneuver around the house with her walker. During this time, my youngest daughter was living at my house and expecting a baby girl soon. A few years back, when she decided not to go away for college like two of her siblings, we transformed the garage area into living quarters for her. It had its own entrance and was set up with a little kitchen with a tile floor, a tiny living area with a sofa across from a bureau and a bed. Eventually, we added a full bathroom as well. It was a perfect setup for my parents.

Before meeting with my dad, I sat down with my daughter and explained to her what could be happening. I asked if she would be willing to move upstairs to her old bedroom so that my parents could live in the "garage." In her beautiful way, she said, *"Of course."*

Back to the story.

I wanted to get to the rehab center a little early and talk with my father. My two older brothers did not live in the area, so I was the one who helped my parents make all their decisions if they asked. When I arrived, I asked my father to come out of the room because I did not want to discuss this in front of my mother.

I asked Dad, "If you think they are going to ask to put her in a nursing home, would you guys want to move in with me?" He looked at me with delight and a sense of relief and said, "We would love that."

We walked into the meeting, and with almost no small talk at all, the social worker plopped a packet of papers down in front of my father and said, "Here is a list of nursing homes." No emotion. No empathy. Just "tada."

The Move

I looked at my dad, then at the social worker.

"They will move in with me," I said.

Mom would stay at the rehab center until we could get everything set up—get all the supplies, a hospital bed, and all the necessary equipment needed to make the transition smooth.

Everything worked out well. We got everything set up, and my nieces arrived just as we were moving my parents into their new space. They helped my father move Mom and assisted my daughter in setting up her new space upstairs.

What a wonderful multigenerational household. My granddaughter had been born by then, so we had four generations living together. I also had a grandson who had been living with me since he was a baby. So now you see, the club sandwich generation.

Getting Settled

My father decided he wanted to sell their house, where they had lived for 53 years. Because my parents spent so much time square dancing, round dancing, and RV traveling, they had not done any updates to the house for at least the past thirty-three years.

The house had bright wallpaper, and some of it was painted. On the main level, the hardwood floors were still in good condition, but the basement floors were very outdated. Additionally, there had been no updates to the laundry room or the powder room. There were so many updates needed to bring the house up to township code.

Who was going to buy this house?

My parents had wonderful neighbors. When it snowed, they would snow-blow their sidewalk and driveway. Many times, they helped with lawn care during the summer. This same neighbor was looking for a house for their grown son and not only offered my father cash for the house but also said they would do all the necessary work to bring the house up to code. Problem solved. The neighbor was a handyman. My father was so grateful.

I spent the next few weekends going into the house and taking out all the items I thought they would want. I brought most of the items to my basement, and the neighbor said he would get rid of anything left in the house. I moved as much as I could in my car, and then my son helped me move the remaining items with a truck rental.

My father never really wanted to go back into the house after Mom's stroke once they moved in with me. I think he felt that part of his life was over and had no desire to return.

My parents loved having the baby in the house, and my daughter never minded taking her in to visit with them. Once the baby could walk, she would visit them multiple times a day by herself. We would all try to have dinner together in the evenings.

My parents moved in at the end of May. My father would never bother me if he could handle any situation. I told him I would help anytime; he just needed to let me know.

First Hospital Visit

One evening, Dad climbed halfway up the stairs in the middle of the night, a bit flustered. I could hear him calling me.

"Sally, can you help? Mom fell, and I can't pick her up." I had no idea how long he had been trying to get her up, but if I had to guess, it had been quite a while.

She was lying on the floor in the middle of the room. My mother did not like using her walker and would always try to walk without it, even though my father constantly reminded her she really needed to use it. Sure enough, she got up to go to the bathroom without her walker and fell.

When I got closer, I realized her leg was awkwardly turned outward. I was certain she had broken her hip.

We called for an ambulance, and when they arrived, the paramedics asked my father if he wanted them to help her back into bed or take her to the hospital. I thought this was a crazy question to ask, given that my father was clearly upset.

In his distressed state, my father was having a hard time making the decision. I calmly told him to look at her leg. Even if we got her into bed, there was no way we would be able to transport her in the morning.

He decided to let them take her to the hospital. She had broken her hip and needed surgery. Eventually, she would need rehab. This time in rehab was a bit different. Not only did they help her get back up and walk with the walker, but they also managed to get her to swallow food again.

YAY! The feeding tube was removed, which was such a relief for my father.

As always seems to be the case, there was more perfect timing within my family. My ex-sister-in-law came for a visit with her partner while my mother was still in the hospital. They were only staying for a few days, and on the day of their planned departure, my mother had some heart trouble.

They called me at work to tell me the doctors had asked them to leave the room, and they did not want to leave my father alone. They were so kind and waited until I could be by my dad's side before they began their 16-hour journey back home. I was so blessed and grateful for their presence. By the time I arrived, Mom's heart event had passed.

Old Man Winter

As winter approached, the temperatures started to fall. Remember, they were living in what used to be a garage. Despite it being well insulated, Mom was always cold.

Now imagine this: Mom would get up and walk to the thermostat, turning the heat up to 90 degrees. My father would get too hot and, sometimes, instead of turning the heat down a bit, he would sleep in his undershirt and shorts.

Unfortunately, the heating bill became very high.

At that time, I enjoyed attending local home shows that featured booths for new kitchens, bathrooms, grouting, gardens, hot tubs, and anything else you could think of for the home. During one show, I saw a booth for a solar panel system and decided to take the plunge and purchase one. Even though it would be an entire year before I saw the difference in my bill, it was a great decision.

My parents did not have a lot of money for retirement, but my father insisted on paying me $300 a month for rent. Throughout their time living with me, I never asked my father for anything, yet he never missed a month. Like clockwork, at the first of the month, my father would hand me a check.

Getting Help

One summer day, when it was 90 degrees outside, I had just gotten home from work when my next-door neighbor stopped by. He wanted to let me know that my father had been outside mowing the lawn in the 90+ degree weather.

"I am afraid something will happen to him," said my concerned neighbor.

My neighbors were the absolute best and were always looking out for my parents. My dad always wanted to help me around the house and would find things he could handle on his own without any complaints.

I remember the very first night they moved in and we all had dinner together. After dinner, my father insisted on washing the dishes. He washed the dishes every single night after that, and anytime any of the grandkids offered to wash the dishes, he would shoo them away. He felt very proud of his job. I think it made him feel better too.

Now, back to the lawn. We had an agreement: he would mow the front yard, and I would mow the backyard. The backyard was much, much bigger than the front, and instead of telling him I didn't want him to mow at all, I told him I was getting tired of mowing the back and would hire someone to mow the entire lawn.

One of my coworkers' husbands did this for a living, and he has been mowing my lawn ever since. My father also liked to go out and shovel the snow. Eventually, the lawn guy would swing by using his snow blower to clear the driveway and sidewalks.

Remember, my parents liked to help out with anything and everything they could get their hands on. One day, I came home from work and found my mother bending over the top of her walker, wiping down the floor in their bathroom. I get it—she just wanted to clean.

I did not want to risk my mother hurting herself again in any way, nor did I want my father to feel obligated to clean either. I decided to hire someone to clean the house.

One day, on the bus I occasionally rode for work, I mentioned to the bus driver that I was looking for someone to come clean the house. Her daughter cleaned houses to supplement her income while attending college, and it worked out perfectly.

My father handled all the scheduling with her and decided he would be the one to pay her. She came every three to four weeks. She was so wonderful to them, and I know he always looked forward to talking to her during her visits.

The Officer and the Swing

The neighborhood loved my parents. Even though my mom couldn't talk, she would smile and wave at everyone. The neighbors across the street were a younger couple with children, and they got along really well with my daughter. Their children would even come over and visit "Grandmom and Grandpop." When their real grandparents visited, they would walk over and spend some time visiting with my parents.

After a few conversations, they realized they had one thing in common—square dancing. They discovered they had danced with some of the same people and had even attended some of the same clubs.

My mother loved to walk outside, but my father could not walk with her because she walked much slower than his back could handle. So, he would let her walk outside by herself.

One day, when I got home from work, my father had quite the story. My mother had gone for her usual walk around the neighborhood and somehow managed to cross a street she didn't cross very often. My dad was sitting in the house when there was a knock at the door. When he opened it, he found a police officer standing there with my mom by his side. They had found her walking aimlessly, and since she couldn't talk, she had a challenging time telling them where she lived.

The officer said she did a lot of pointing, and somehow they ended up in the area where my parents used to live, which was about 20 minutes away. The officer made his way back to where they picked her up, and finally, she was able to point out the house where she lived now. The officer asked my father if he could take a picture of Mom to keep in their database in case this happened again. My father completely agreed and decided to get Mom a bracelet with her name, address, and phone number on it. WHEW! What a day for my dad!

On another occasion, I came home and Mom was not in her room. I asked my dad where she was, and he said she was walking in the backyard. There was a swing set in the back for the grandkids, and my mother enjoyed swinging on it too. The neighbors would mention how much joy they had watching her swing freely from time to time.

I walked into the backyard and quickly noticed she was lying on the ground. I wasn't sure if she was lying there on purpose or if she had fallen. My guess was that she had fallen. My father had no idea how long she had been out there or lying with her back flat on the ground. I could tell she was upset because she couldn't move or call for help.

My father and I were not able to lift her because she was "dead weight." I went to another neighbor's house across the street who was home. As I was knocking on his door, another neighbor from down the street was driving by, and I flagged him down. My father brought the wheelchair up from the basement. We had this for my mother when my father took her to appointments that required a lot of walking. I could tell she had not broken anything, so the neighbors were able to lift her up and put her in the wheelchair. We got her safely back in the house. I don't think she ever walked out back after that.

The Dog & Another Person in the House

One of my grandsons had lived with me from the time he was little. Every summer, he looked forward to going to camp. We had decided that when he came back from camp, we would get a dog. This was the spring after my parents moved in with us. He and I went to the SPCA and found Sammie, the dog.

Once we got home, Sammie attached himself to my mother and was always by her side. Of course, she also fed Sammie anything we were eating at dinner. Sammie never ate his food from the dog bowl, which frustrated my father immensely. Sammie also liked to run after squirrels, so we could never let my mother take him for a walk. We let Sammie run around in the fenced backyard, but with my mother's slow pace, we were always afraid the dog would pull her down.

Now, back to my grandson. His father had been in and out of jail due to poor choices. At one point, he had been in a halfway house and wanted my grandson and me to come visit. We had visited him while he was in the county prison years before. During our visit, his father mentioned that if he didn't have a place to live after the halfway house, he would have to return to jail. My grandson and I just looked at each other. When we got home, we talked about it, and my grandson, with his big heart, asked if his dad could live with us. I discussed it with my parents. By then, my daughter was no longer living in the house, so we had two extra bedrooms upstairs. I let his father know he was welcome to stay with us. Little did we know what that entailed.

He had a parole officer who needed to meet with my father and me before he could move in. We couldn't have any guns in the house, which we didn't own anyway, but my grandson had a paintball gun, so we took that out of the house just to be sure.

During the meeting, the parole officer told us all the rules his client needed to follow. He had to be in by nine o'clock in the evening. The parole officer also informed us that he could come anytime to visit and check on his client. He said that if he couldn't get in the house, he would need to break down the door. We hoped that wouldn't happen, so we agreed to let him stay with us and signed the paperwork.

He followed all the rules and even got a job within walking distance. He eventually bought a car and got a different job. My father and mother saw him more often than I did. Since my grandson was in school, he didn't see him much either. The father would get home in time for his curfew.

About eight or nine months into his stay with us, I noticed one evening that he did not come in by his curfew. He had also been leaving for work by four-thirty in the morning, so I rarely saw him. That morning, his car was still parked by the curb. When I got home from work, the car wasn't there. I asked my grandson if he had seen his dad that morning before he left for school. He said no, but his car was still there. That evening, when the father still hadn't come home, I asked my dad if he had seen him.

My parents loved to sit in their room during the day. Once they were up and about, they would open the shade and watch all that was going on outside the house. My father said he saw my grandson's father pull his car into the driveway and go in and out of the house carrying stuff. My father said he never came and talked to him.

When I didn't see his car the following morning, I decided to look in the room. It was completely empty except for trash. For some reason, I decided to look under the mattress, and there I found his wallet. I kept it just in case my grandson would ever want it. He did not say goodbye to his son or my parents.

I called the parole officer and left a message to let him know. It took a couple of weeks, but finally, the parole officer got back to me. Apparently, the parole officer had been to the house one day, and the father had told him he was moving to Ohio and getting married. Since then, none of us have heard from him.

Brotherhood

My father had two brothers. After my mother had her stroke, he would only go places if she could go with him. One of his brothers lived in another state. When my father turned ninety, both his brothers, their children, and the rest of the family came to celebrate. The brother who lived out of state would call him to talk. He called on the house phone because my father could hear better from that phone, even though I had gotten him a cell phone for when he went out. As soon as I heard my uncle's voice, I would say hello and then get my father on the phone. We had extensions in our rooms and the kitchen.

One call, my uncle asked to speak to me first. He wanted to tell me that he had been diagnosed with lung cancer and asked if he should tell my father. I said absolutely yes.

My father was very stoic and preferred to know something rather than not. My father wanted to visit but would not leave my mother, so he asked me to go. I flew there and spent a weekend with my aunt and uncle and then flew back. I was able to see one of my brothers, who lived about a half hour from my aunt and uncle, and we both visited them together.

Within six weeks, my uncle passed away. My father was very sad about this and then asked me to go to the funeral to represent him and my mother, which I did. I flew in again for the funeral, and my brother and I met up and went to the funeral together.

2009

Three years after my parents moved in, the daughter who had lived with us announced that she was expecting her second child. She visited my mother and father almost daily, or at least four to five times a week. This was exciting news for all of us.

My mother only had one sister. She had asked me to sign papers to help her with her checkbooks and paperwork and to make any necessary medical decisions. She had no children, and her husband had passed away just a few years after they got married. I adored my aunt. She had moved to a lifecare community where she was having fun, socializing, and would be taken care of if she became ill.

That spring, my aunt fell and broke her hip. She had surgery and rehab and was able to return to her community, but she moved to the facility where she had nursing services. My daughter often visited my aunt with her own daughter. My father would take my mother, and they spent as much time as they could visiting my aunt and keeping her company.

One morning near my daughter's due date, she must have sensed she was going into labor. Her first labor and delivery had been very quick. She asked to stay at my house and had her daughter stay with her grandfather. That morning, she told her husband to go to work and then called me into the room. I called her husband right away and said he needed to come back immediately as my daughter was in labor. We went to the hospital, and again she had a quick delivery.

After her son was born, her daughter came to the hospital. Once she visited her new brother, she came home with me. My father, mother, and I, along with my granddaughter, visited my aunt because my granddaughter liked to see her. While we were there, my aunt was not responding very well. My granddaughter sat next to her, rubbing her head and telling her all about her new baby brother. That same evening, I received a call just before midnight that my aunt had passed away. September 18, 2009—the circle of life.

Day to Day

My father always wanted to leave the house every day. He would take my mother and go to the supermarket and buy a few items. He would get my mother's prescriptions filled or they would go out for lunch. He had stopped driving in the dark quite a while before this.

They would also meet their friends for lunch at a local restaurant or visit his other brother. His brother would sometimes come and visit them at the house. I remember one visit when his brother was still driving, they said the worst thing that could happen is to lose their driver's license and not have the independence to get around. Soon after this conversation his brother did indeed have to stop driving. He had been living with one of his children and moved to a veteran's community. This was about a little less than an hour drive from our house. It was a little too long for my father to drive. When my parents wanted to see him we started going together so I could drive. My uncle liked corned beef sandwiches and my mother liked lox and bagel. So, before we would go visit, I would head out to the local delicatessen and get all that we wanted for lunch along with potato salad and rye bread, pickles and something to drink and we would have our "picnic" with him in one of the small cafeteria areas. I know my parents always looked forward to seeing him. We were also able to celebrate my uncle's 90th birthday at the veteran's center with all of his family.

My father would also take my mother to all of her appointments. She was going to physical therapy and occupational therapy. She would have blood work done once a month. They also tried speech therapy. The therapist was able to get a special computer in which she hoped to teach my mother to use the computer to communicate. Due to the stroke, she was never able to pick up the concept of looking at the computer and pointing to what she wanted. My father was disappointed. There were times that this became very frustrating for the both of them.

As time passed my parents were very comfortable with their daily schedule. By the time they would get up, washed and dressed and had their breakfast it would be about eleven o'clock in the morning. They would have lunch around two o'clock and be ready to eat whenever I had dinner ready to serve.

One morning after 8:00 am and they weren't up yet, the dog started barking and there was a knock on the door. It was the police again. This time my grandson had been hit by a car on his way to school. He would ride his bike every morning to school. He was under the car but awake and aware.He gave the police his address and they came looking for a phone number since at the time I had guardianship. There was a bulletin board in my parents room and I kept a card pinned on with my phone number if my father ever needed me. They called me when I was already on my way to the scene. Luckily, a bystander had kneeled down to talk to my grandson and he told them where I worked and the person called my work and I got the message and was on my way. Scary for all of us. He was flown to the Children's Hospital of Philadelphia and discharged that afternoon.

Another day, my father told me the police had stopped by the house. Apparently there was a robbery suspect who drove a car the same color and make as my father's and someone saw his car in the driveway and reported it to the police. I think after some conversation with my father the police realized he wasn't the suspect.

One of the items that we brought from their house was a treadmill. My mother loved walking on this. She would be able to somehow communicate to my father that she wanted to walk. He would set it all up for her and once she was on it would set it on the lowest number and my mother would walk for twenty minutes. She wore out the soles of a few pairs of sneakers because she could not lift her one foot as well and it would drag on the treadmill. When she couldn't use the treadmill anymore, she wanted to continue to do another form of exercise. Now they had received lots of catalogs in the mail. My mother was able to point to things she wanted my father to order. My mother found a bicycle peddler that she could use while sitting on the edge of her bed. My father ordered anything she wanted from the catalogs. She would sit and pedal for twenty minutes.

At one point my mother began having trouble walking up the one step to get into the kitchen. It was an eight-inch step. My father measured the area and told me what size pieces of wood to buy and he would build a four-inch step. When I went to the local home improvement store and started asking the employee to cut each piece of wood to a certain size, he asked me what I was getting it for. I explained that my mother could no longer get up the one step into the kitchen and we were making it so that she could only go up four inches and it would also be the width of the walker. The employee went and got an electric screwdriver and built the step right there for me. I was so grateful. Before I left the store, I asked how I could let the company know. I did call as soon as I went into my car as I had made sure I had his name.

Getting Tired

It was becoming increasingly difficult for my father to help my mother with her daily activities. One day, I came home and he told me they both had fallen after her shower, but he had managed to get them both up without any injuries.

When they first moved in, we had met Sharon, who was helping another couple as a home health aide. We met her again the following year, and she told us the couple she had been caring for had passed away. She gave us her information, and I talked to my father about calling her. We decided to reach out to her, and she started coming two to three times a week to help my mother shower. She was such a blessing. With her help, we were able to keep my mother at home and avoid moving her to a nursing home.

Despite Sharon's assistance, it was still becoming more difficult for my father to assist my mother. Then one day, my mother just couldn't get out of bed. We were supposed to visit my uncle that day. Between the two of us, we managed to get my mother into a wheelchair and to the car, bringing her to the emergency room. That was the last time she was in the house.

My mother was admitted to the hospital for a week as the doctors tried to figure out what had happened. There was no clear diagnosis. She was then sent to a rehabilitation center. My father was not happy with this facility, but he visited her every day and stayed all day. Two days later, she slumped over while sitting up in a chair in her room. They called an ambulance, and she was transported back to the hospital.

Again, there was no clear diagnosis.

When they wanted to discharge her again to a rehab center, my father insisted he did not like the previous one. The hospital social worker helped him find another facility that was covered by her insurance and not too far from the house. She stayed there, and within two months, she was able to walk again with her walker, though much slower and less steady. She needed to be discharged, but my father knew he could no longer handle her daily care at home.

Celebration of Love

My father realized he needed help with his finances. We met with an elder lawyer who helped my father set up a trust to ensure my mother would have money for her care in case something happened to him. During this time, he and I also made sure all the necessary paperwork was done for him in case he became ill or disabled. He was able to get her into an assisted living facility.

Even though my mother couldn't speak, we still believed she understood what was happening. We decorated her room, and I still have the butterfly that hung on her door. She participated in all the activities, and my father had lunch and dinner with her every day. He would then come home, watch the Phillies play, go to sleep, and get up the next day to spend the day with her. He never missed a day.

One early morning, after she had been there for about two months, we got a call that she had tried to get out of bed herself and had fallen, breaking her hip. This was devastating. Back to the hospital, back to surgery, and back to rehab. We managed to get her back into the rehab facility my father was comfortable with and that was not too far from the house. However, her recovery was not as good as it had been with the last broken hip. She had more trouble moving and was unable to get up from the chair on her own. Eventually, the facility said they could no longer keep her in the rehab section, and my father decided to move her to the nursing home side of the facility. She had two other roommates, and her insurance covered most of the expenses.

In June 2013, we were able to use one of their conference rooms to celebrate my parents' 65th wedding anniversary. It was wonderful to have a few family members join us. Right after the celebration, I left for a conference I had signed up for months before. My grandson accompanied me, and we planned to attend the conference and take a cruise to Alaska.

A week after our return, my mother developed a severe case of diarrhea and had to be moved to an isolation room. My father and I knew things were not looking good. We decided to ask for hospice help. We only had three days, but they were very helpful to my father. On Sunday morning, we got a call that she was breathing very slowly and that we should come in to sit with her. The hospice nurse stopped in and explained the type of breathing we might see and that we could ask for medication from the nursing staff. She also said we would know when the last moment of her life was near.

She began breathing much slower, making unusual sounds late in the afternoon. I could see this really bothered my father, so I asked the nurse to bring the medication hospice had suggested. The nurse didn't come right away.

As I returned to the room, I looked into my mother's eyes, and I showed my father. We knew.

I went out into the hall to get the nurse, and not just one, but two nurses came. They stayed with us until she took her last breath, until she transitioned. This was very comforting.

It was July 20, 2013.

My mother and father had decided about twenty years before that they would both like to be cremated. They had paid all the expenses over time and carried the cremation card in their wallets. As soon as my mother passed, I called both of my brothers. We had been keeping them updated all along. My father pulled out his wallet and said we needed to call the crematory right away, as they had been instructed. I told him we could wait a little, but he insisted.

I called and left a message, and the answering service said someone would call us back shortly. Five minutes later, the phone rang, and I answered, confused because it wasn't the service but my cousin calling to let us know she had heard about my mother from my brother. We were grateful my brother thought to call the cousins, but I was momentarily confused, thinking it was the cremation people. They did call back a few minutes later and said they would come and get my mother's body. We called my children, and one came with her husband to pack all of my mother's belongings from her regular room. I asked my father if he was ready to go home.

My father did not want to leave. He wanted to wait.

The nurses prepared her body, and we waited in the lounge by the front door. When the man arrived, my father said we would accompany him to the room with the gurney. My father and I helped him move her to the gurney and zip up the bag. We walked to the car with her body.

Once she was in the car, my father said, *"Okay, I am ready to go home now."*

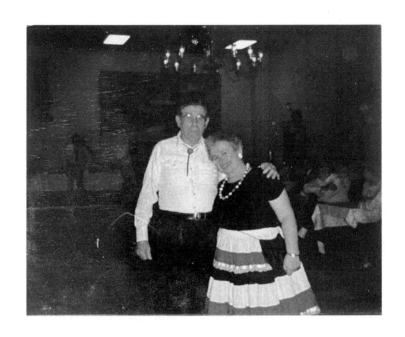

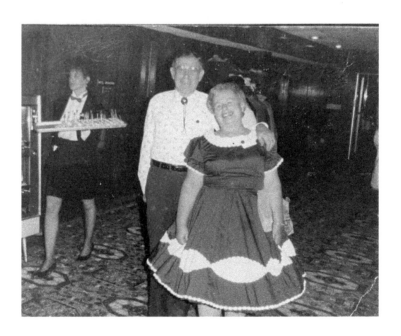

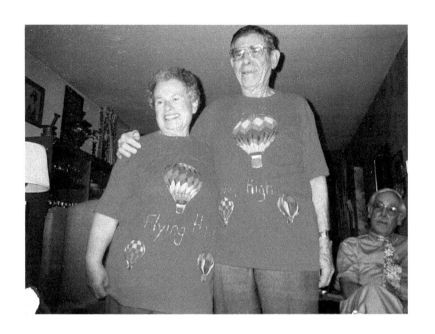

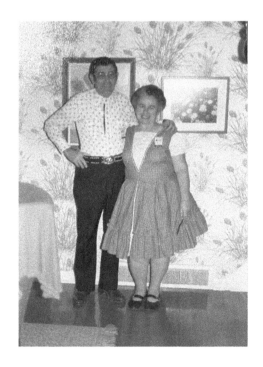

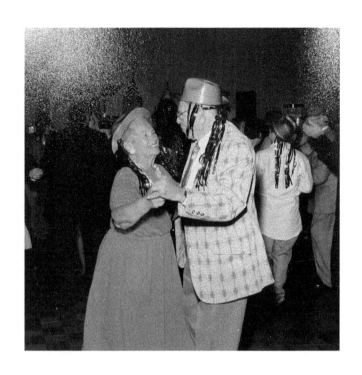

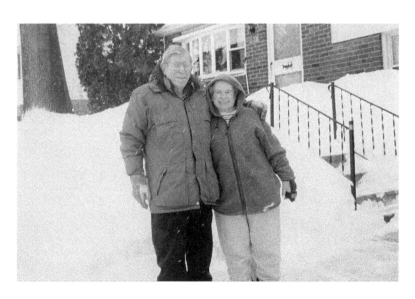

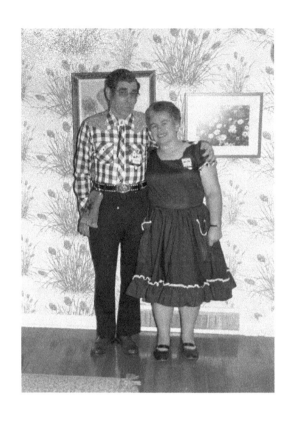

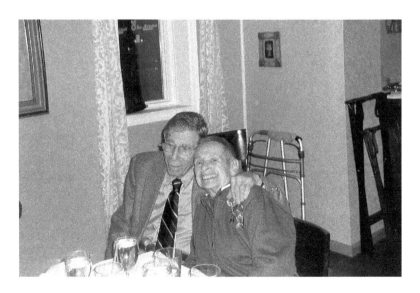

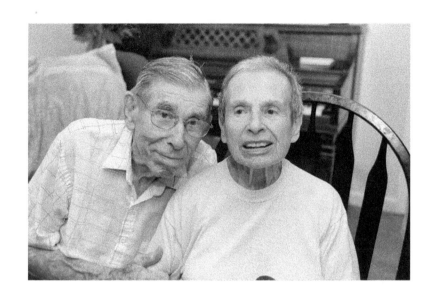

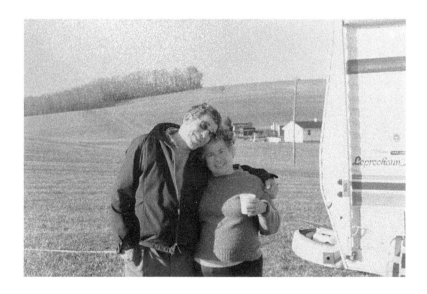

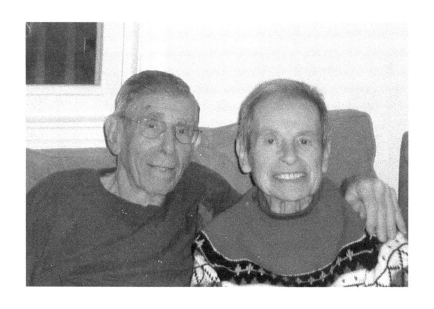

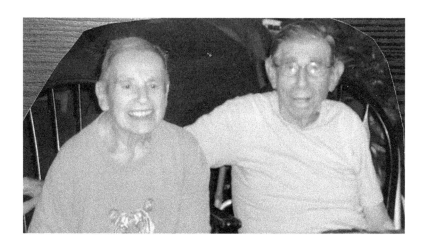

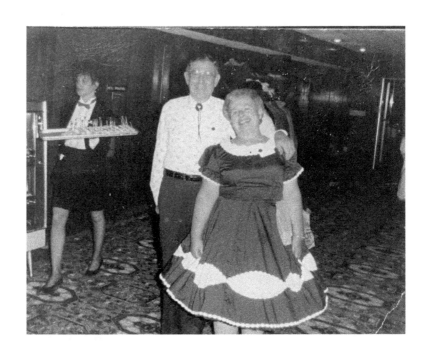

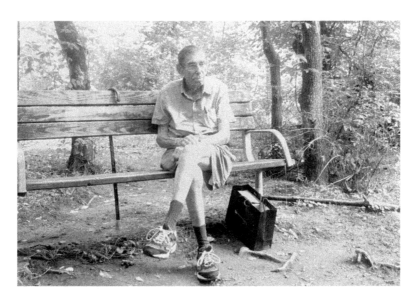

Silent Memories

My father wanted to have a memorial service for my mother. So, first, we needed to decide on a place and a date. He wanted a Rabbi to lead the service. The life celebration center he chose was wonderful. They worked with him to set the date, arrange the announcement in the newspaper, and secure a compassionate Rabbi.

Another little backstory for you.

My parents had been a host family for a few people from the International House at the University of Pennsylvania. The last one was when I was thirteen, and he was from India, studying for his doctorate degree. In fact, I later found his thesis and sent it to his daughter. When the exchange student met me and found out I was not engaged, he asked if he could bring his two daughters to America and live with us until he got settled. They were nine and eleven years old at that time. They lived in bunk beds in our basement for a year and are now my "sisters."

Back to the service.

One of the sisters had since passed, but the other one flew in from the West Coast to join us. Their father had passed away a number of years before. Not only did she fly in, but she also sent my brother his fare so he could come as well. My older brother and his wife were able to attend and stayed for a week.

The service was beautiful. Most of the family and some of their friends attended, as well as many people from the square dance organization they had belonged to for many years.

Once the service was over and everyone went home, my father wanted to place my mother's ashes where they had both agreed to. He didn't want to go with anyone but me.

It was a beautiful Sunday afternoon in a park by a running creek and a small waterfall. We didn't know if we were allowed to do this or not and hadn't asked anyone, but we were doing it. This was a place they both loved to walk to from their house. There was a bench by the water in the shade. No matter how hot it was outside, that area was always cool. They would sit, have conversations, and enjoy nature.

When my father and I arrived, there was a young man fishing with his son. We decided we would just sit and enjoy the area if other people were there. They left shortly after we arrived.

My father was very organized. He brought the ashes in the box they came in and had a cup so we could take out some ashes at a time and not dump the whole box at once. Over the next hour and a half, we slowly placed the ashes in the water and along the trees and roots by the creek. My father had his own conversations with my mother while sitting there.

Once we were done, we sat in silence and reflected on my mother's life.

It was a very spiritual experience.

Life without Mom

After my mother's passing, my father had to adjust to being home every day without having to drive back and forth somewhere. He felt sad but got up every day and made do with his life. He mentioned that most of his friends had already passed away, and those who were still alive he couldn't visit anymore. My youngest daughter continued to visit him with her children, and he always looked forward to their visits.

My father missed taking my mother out every day and visiting her every day. He didn't want to eat out alone, so almost every day, we went out for dinner. I got tired of going to the same places and eating the same food, so I asked everyone I would meet about different restaurants and diners they liked. We began to explore the area and different restaurants and diners. Occasionally I rode the bus for work and I would ask the drivers about places to eat, and they made many suggestions. I kept a little book in my purse and wrote down everyone's favorite places.

In October 2013, after my mother passed away, we celebrated my uncle's 90th birthday with him and all his family. Shortly after those celebrations, he passed away. Now, my father, being the oldest sibling, was the only one still alive.

Another backstory for you.

My parents had a unique relationship with my older brother. I probably don't know most of what happened. What I do know is that when he was still in high school, he decided to leave for one weekend without telling them where he was going or why. He returned and graduated from high school. He went to a technical school and learned printing. He moved out west and did not contact them for a long time. When I graduated from college

(1981), they wanted me to reach out to him. Eventually, after calling a few people, I got him on the phone. He asked how I got his number, which didn't really require an answer since I was talking to him, but he said, *"I am looking for myself and please do not contact me again."* I responded by saying, *"When you find yourself, please give us a call."* My parents did not hear from him again until about 20 years later.

One Thanksgiving before mom passed, she asked my son to go on the computer and see how many MGs he could find in California. He found 20 with phone numbers. I just started calling down the list, saying I was looking for MG who graduated from my high school. The fourth call was my brother.

He had just married a wonderful woman who told us she had been trying to convince him to get in contact with us again. My parents were very relieved and happy to have him back in their lives and, luckily. he and his wife managed to visit a few times over the years before my mother passed on.

Back to life without mom.

In December 2013, after my mother's service, I received a call from my brother's wife. My brother had not been feeling well, and she had to take him to the hospital. They didn't know what was wrong with him. When she brought him home the first time, he could hardly move and had turned yellow. Their homeopathic doctor advised her to bring him back to the hospital. The local hospital transferred him to a big teaching hospital in the city.

My brother was an extremely loving person and had written a couple of books on spirituality. According to my sister-in-law, who is also very loving, he knew he was dying by the end of February, and she managed to get him home on hospice. She said he couldn't move, and she worked very hard to keep him comfortable. He passed away in her arms at home. This was very hard for my father, especially when she sent a picture of the two of them resting comfortably in bed before he passed away. She had a memorial service for him in California and, two weeks later, came to visit us. We were very grateful as she held a service in our house that we could participate in and sang the songs he loved. This was another loss my father had to endure. He often told me that this was one of the hardest things about getting older.

Sammie the Dog

Sammie, our dog, was still around, always greeting my father. Sammie could no longer sleep with my mother but stayed close to my father after her passing. My father would go out and buy the dog his food and treats. One day, Sammie came in from the backyard limping badly. My father took him to the vet, and Sammie needed an operation on his leg, which he recovered from. My father would let the dog in and out of the back door to run around and use the yard as needed.

After the operation, my father noticed that Sammie was getting up more frequently to go outside but wasn't peeing much each time. He took the dog back to the vet, and it was discovered that Sammie had a tumor and had been losing weight. My father decided to forgo further treatment and asked the vet to put the dog to sleep.

My father didn't want to be with the dog when this happened. I took two of my grandchildren to spend time with Sammie the night before. The next day, my oldest grandson also wanted to see the dog. He met me at the vet, said his good-bye but didn't want to stay in the room with Sammie while she was put to sleep. I sat with Sammie and the vet while she took her last breath in the fall of 2014.

Laughter & the Winter Blues

At this time, I had 10 grandchildren, and my father had 11 great-grandchildren. My niece was planning to visit that Thanksgiving with her son and my father was really looking forward to their visit, as he had enjoyed their visit the year before. They stayed for a few days, and the visiting grandson would spend lots of time with my dad and as it turns out, they entertained one another with lots of laughter and just enjoying the company of the other.

A few days after they left, my father noticed blisters on his hands. As I mentioned before, he was not one to complain or go to the doctor much. He would go to his yearly physicals because the insurance company would call and ask him to go. During his physical in December, when he turned 96, he passed his physical and was cleared to drive. When he received his new license, he said, *"This one is good until I am one hundred years old. I don't think I will renew it after that."*

At one of the doctor's visits, my father mentioned that he was getting old and the doctor told him he had to live another eight years since still had eight years left on his mortgage. My father had a good laugh at that.

When the blisters started, my father didn't say much about them. As they continued, he said they felt better when he popped them. I was afraid of infection, so I made sure he had alcohol pads to clean whatever pin he was using. The blisters weren't getting better, but he didn't want to go to the doctor. One day in December 2014, he told me he had stopped driving because his hands were too sore, and he was afraid he would lose control of the steering wheel. This made him feel sad and depressed.

On Christmas Eve, he became so uncomfortable that he agreed to let me take him to see his doctor. By then, the blisters were on his hands and feet. The doctor gave him some medication. I was lucky to be off from work at this time. Every morning, I would come down and help him with his blisters. It would take me at least two hours daily to help him get comfortable and dress all the blisters. On New Year's Eve, he was in more pain, so we went back to the doctor, who prescribed even stronger pain medication.

The morning after the winter holiday break, I went down to see him before I left for work. I had warned him it would be early. One of his legs looked very red, like it could be an infection. I wanted to take him to the hospital right away but he insisted that go to work and come back later in the morning because wanted to get up, wash his body, and eat his breakfast to stick to his routine of getting washed, dressed, and eating by 11 o'clock every morning.

I ended up taking a half-day from work and took him to the emergency room. We shared with the staff about him seeing the doctor twice in December. The ER doctor thought it was an infection, but after the blood tests came back, the doctor said it wasn't an infection but did state that it was some kind of skin problem and arranged for us to see a dermatologist the next morning.

It is very hard to get an appointment with a dermatologist, and this one told us he wasn't taking any new patients but would fit us in since the emergency room doctor called him. He was wonderful with my father and very patient. On the first day, we saw him at 8 o'clock in the morning as that was the only time he would see us. My father managed to break out of his routine and get ready. After that, the doctor agreed to see him at the end of the day around four in the afternoon.

After examining my father, the doctor left the room and said he would be back to do a biopsy. The nurse came in, and my father signed the papers. When the doctor returned, he took biopsies from my father's forehead, cheek, and three blisters on his legs. My father didn't understand why his face was being biopsied when he came in about the blisters. The doctor believed the other spots looked cancerous. My father said he had those spots for years and didn't want them removed.

The results came back, and the doctor had us come back in. My father was diagnosed with an autoimmune skin disease and the doctor explained that treating this disease was challenging for a 57 year-old, and even more challenging for a 97 year-old. The doctor also wanted to remove the lesion on my father's cheek because it was skin cancer, which he was able to remove during our visit. He told my father the one on his forehead was melanoma, and he would need to see a specialist as well as a specialist for the skin problem.

Unbearable Pain

My father was having trouble sitting for long periods due to pain and blisters all over his body. On the way home from the appointment, we picked up all the prescriptions. Some of the creams were over two hundred dollars, and my father's insurance did not cover medication. My father didn't want to go to any of the appointments, but I set them up anyway because the dermatologist's office would call and ask when they were scheduled. The specialist for the melanoma said he would need to sit for four hours to do the procedure. My father expressed to me that he knew he could not do it.

Through January and into February, he was unable to be mobile due to the pain. It would take me about two to three hours daily to change all the dressings. The blisters covered his legs and had started on his chest, back, and stomach. He began using a bedside commode since his feet were very sore, and he couldn't bear to walk to the bathroom. We had many supplies saved from my mother's care so he would use my mother's walker to help him stand up. My daughter would stop by every day to check on him. By then, he allowed me to stay home from work occasionally. He was afraid to take the pain medication because of how it made him feel. One day, he told me he had taken the pain medication, made it to the bathroom, but had to crawl back to bed, so he just didn't want to take it anymore.

One of my daughters called her siblings, saying she thought their *"Saba"*, which was their nickname for my dad instead of calling him grandpa, and she requested they all come to visit one weekend in January. By then, we were eating in his room because he could not walk far, and was definitely not able to use the steps into the kitchen.

When they all came, two of my sons-in-law helped him in the wheelchair and lifted it up the one step into the dining room. We were all able to eat together that day. He, with 10 of his great-grandchildren, me, and four of his grandchildren. The 11th grandchild had already visited back in November.

Because the pain was so bad, I would come down in the morning, and he would tell me all kinds of ways he was going to end his life. One morning, he said he wanted a tube to attach to the car's exhaust pipe. I pointed out that he couldn't even walk to the car. He laughed out loud as he knew he couldn't get to the door. Then another morning, he said he was going to put the folding chair outside and sit in the freezing temperatures. The doctor was not able to help us find any solutions for his unbearable pain, both physically and mentally.

My father and I talked about possibly moving him to rehab to get the pain and dressing changes under control for his comfort and well-being.

He agreed, and since his insurance was different from my mother's. He did not have to be in the hospital for three days for his insurance to kick in; he just needed to come from a hospital setting. He wanted me to call the place my mother had been in to see if they had a bed available. They did have a rehab bed available which gave him the courage to see if this would help his pain. I took him to the emergency room and the doctor saw how much pain he was in and wanted to admit him. My father did not want to stay in the hospital and we shared what we knew about the rehab center, and the doctor was okay with that. With slow steps and hopefulness, I took him to the rehab center with paperwork from the hospital.

No More Pain

The rehab had a system for dressing changes, and he was initially on the team that did the treatment in the middle of the night. I stayed the first night with him until it was done. He said he would not allow them to do it without me there. At our insistence, they changed him to the day schedule. It took two nurses over an hour to do his complete dressing changes. The nurse would give him pain medication before each change, but he still cried every time it happened. When not undergoing dressing changes, he enjoyed being there. There was always someone stopping in to talk to him as he was very pleasant and always had a joke to tell.

A physical therapist worked with him to keep his strength up, and an occupational therapist helped him find the best utensils to eat with since his hands hurt so much. The nurses requested a speech therapist to work with him, because he always had trouble swallowing big pills or pieces of food. At first, he would cut his pills in half before he could swallow them, eventually I would take over.

I could see that he was eating less and less. During this time, there was a lot of snow and a holiday, so I was able to spend more time with him. My daughter was with us during one of his dressing changes and she witnessed how much pain and suffering he would endure. I think he knew deep down he could not continue suffering for much longer and we knew too.

On Friday, February 20, I took a half-day off work to spend the whole afternoon with him. He had called me before I arrived to let me know he was in a lot of pain. The nurses finally gave him his pain medication and we had a wonderful afternoon. He joked with the physical therapist, had an interesting conversation with the speech therapist, occupational therapist, and social worker. Everyone always enjoyed his company. He had a caring way about him and continued to tell jokes.

His dressing changes were becoming so painful for me to watch. When it was finished and the nurses had left, he looked at me and said, *"I have had enough. I can't do this anymore."*

We spoke about his wish to live to be one hundred. He said that was no longer important. I said good night to him as the sun went down, he gave me a kiss and hug and he told me he loved me. I told him I loved him too and would see him in the morning.

The weather report for the weekend was going to be a doozy winter storm, so when I got home, I packed extra clothes, knowing I wouldn't be able to drive home. I had already planned to stay with him for the weekend. When I arrived at his room the next morning, he didn't respond to my greeting. I saw that he was all pulled up in bed and looked comfortable. I asked the aide if he flinched or made a grimace when they moved him, and the aide said no. I knew then he had made up his mind that he was ready to move on.

I called all my children, my brother, my sister-in-law, and my cousin to let them know he was no longer responding. I was supposed to meet my friend and I called her because I wasn't going to be able to go. She ended up coming to sit with me while I sat with my dad. All the kids and grandkids who were nearby stopped in, as well as my cousin and his wife.

Since he wasn't responding, I told the staff that I didn't want him moved. My friend suggested initiating hospice, which was a wonderful idea. They put him on pain medication every two hours and let him rest. I stayed overnight in his room, and by Sunday, his breathing became much shallower. I just sat with him, talked to him, and rested. By the afternoon, he was still breathing but more slowly. I thought he must be holding on for something.

I stood by him, put my hand on his chest, and said out loud, *"Dad, everything is okay here. All the grandkids stopped in yesterday, as well as my cousin, and they said they would take care of me."* I knew he was worried about that.

I gave him a kiss and said, *"Just rest now, and I will be fine."* Then his breaths became very slow. I called the nurse from the hallway and she sent in another nurse who sat with me until he took his last breath.

It was February 22, 2015.

Of course, I had to call my brother and sister-in-law to let them know. Then I called the cremation society right away. I remember my dad saying, *"Don't forget to call them as soon as I pass."*

The aide came in and gently washed him and changed the sheets. I packed his things in a bag and waited. When the cremation person arrived, he mentioned that I looked familiar. I reminded him that we had helped with my mother, and now I was going to help with my father.

Together Again

This time, I was on my own making the service arrangements and meeting with everyone, but it wasn't hard as I just followed everything we had done for my mother. I even managed to secure the same compassionate Rabbi. My sister-in-law and brother were able to be there. My other "sister" couldn't attend this time. My father's two friends, as well as family members and people from the square dance club, attended the memorial service.

Once the service was finished and everyone left, I knew I wanted to place his ashes with my mother's. When we had gone to the park before, I had taken many pictures to remember where to go. Once I received the ashes, I had no trouble finding the spot. This time, I was alone. When I first arrived, there were some people there, and I just said hello and quietly sat on the bench. Once they left, I put my father's ashes in the same spots as my mother's. At one point, I thought I heard people walking, but thankfully, no one came close. I had time to be by myself and think about how my mother and father were together again, hopefully enjoying each other's company.

It was, again, a very spiritual experience.

This is what it was like having my parents live with me and enjoy the generations together.

Back to Dancing

By now, I still wanted to dance but didn't want to go far because I was still working full-time. The only dancing nearby was square dancing, so I signed up.

It's now the spring of 2016. I have had four weeks of square-dancing lessons. My neighbor across the street was visiting and working on his daughter's flower gardens. I told him about square dancing, and he said he had just attended a convention with a thousand square dancers. He asked if I had learned certain steps already. Some I recognized, and some I did not. That evening, after talking to him, I decided to write this.

Would you believe I am square dancing!

I feel blessed to have had my mother live with me for seven years and my father for eight and a half years.

Have the Conversation

Their retirements and finances were never a conversation we had. My parents bought a recreational vehicle after I had graduated from college, got married, and moved out of the house. They went on many trips with the RV. They liked to go to Elder Hostels, bike, and square dance. They did this for many many years.

My father told me they had paid off their mortgage as soon as they could, so they didn't have to worry about the house. I had never really thought about their future. I had two brothers living in other states, so this discussion never happened.

So why the book?

I wanted to share about having a multigenerational household and to make sure that if you are an adult with living parents, you become aware of many things that can make your life easier and less stressful for everyone involved, allowing you to enjoy the present moment.

If your children are grown and have graduated from high school and possibly college, have entered the workforce or armed services, or maybe are still living with you, and your parents are still alive and doing well, it might be a good idea to have the conversations about their finances, future, and health care decisions.

Some would suggest you do. Some parents would be willing to have this discussion, while others might not want to because they like to keep this part of their life private.

My parents decided 20 years before that they wanted to be cremated when they passed. They found out the details, paid it off over time, and each carried a card with them in their wallets.

They also decided where they wanted their ashes to be placed. I didn't know about this until my mother had her stroke, and my father told me. My mother had a living will, but my father did not.

They had thought about what decisions they wanted to be made about their health care if something happened to them physically. My father knew he needed to get his wishes in writing. They considered this when they were well and very active. Once my mother had her stroke, my father decided to go to an elder care lawyer to figure out what else they needed.

A lot of care for the elderly also depends on how much money they have "in the bank." If they only have their health insurance, there are places that will take patients but only with certain health issues. Others may be able to live in a life care retirement community and have their health care needs met.

And, with that, have conversations with your parents about their finances, future, and health care decisions.

My Advice to You

Disclaimer:I am not a lawyer, nor do I profess to be one. You should be aware of and investigate all the options, whether you are the elder person or a family member, to understand what exists before a medical crisis or death happens. Once you have all of this together, sit down with your family or family members and review it every few years, or sooner, depending on your situation.

Here is what I recommend you discuss with a family member, and know where to find the information:

- Will
- Power of Attorney
- Medical Power of Attorney
- Living Will
- Consent for Release of Information
- Personal Medical History
- Insurance Information
- Long-term Care Insurance Policy
- Out-of-Hospital Do Not Resuscitate
- Revocable Living Trust
- Financial Documents
- Veteran's Benefits – Military Records
- Bank Accounts, Pensions, Tax Returns, Savings Books
- Deeds on All Properties
- Vehicle Titles
- Loans and Debts – Credit Card Accounts
- Passwords to Access Phone Messages
- Online Usernames and Passwords
- End of Life Instructions (if not in your will)
- Marriage License, Divorce Papers
- Birth Certificate
- Organ Donor Card
- Safety Deposit Box
- Driver's License
- Social Security Number
- Cremation Information
- Burial Information
- Pension Information
- Any Letters of Instruction

Most importantly, TAKE CARE OF YOURSELF! Whether you are the elder or the caregiver, it is essential to maintain your well-being. If you are too tired, worn down, or not eating healthy, you can't be at your best.

Here are a few ways to take care of yourself. Many of these you can define in your own way and add what suits you:

- Care for Your Mental and Emotional Wellbeing
- Have a Good Attitude
- Ask for What You Need
- Educate Yourself
- See a Doctor as Needed – Don't Put It Off
- Get Enough Sleep
- Eat Healthy (more fruits and vegetables)
- Exercise – Do Whatever You Can
- Have a Social Support Network
- Keep Busy – Volunteer – Do What You Love
- Be Kind
- Hydrate – Drink Plenty of Water
- Take Care of Your Personal Needs
- Wear Clothes That Make You Feel Good
- Meditate or Find Other Ways to Relax
- Be Positive
- Do Something You Enjoy Every Day
- Laugh
- Cultivate a Routine
- Get a Pet if You Can
- Write – Keep a Journal
- Be Creative
- Read – Go to the Library – Read Online
- Make Time for Play
- Go Outside
- Stress Less
- Be Happy
- Shop
- Learn Something New
- Love Your Loved Ones
- Enjoy Life

- Find the Positive in Every Situation
- Enjoy the Moments
- Find Moments to Be Grateful
- Cry When You Need To
- Communicate Your Needs
- Consider Hiring Help
- Use Online Resources

Be Aware of:

- Time Demands
- Emotional Strains
- Guilt Feelings
- Financial Strain
- Loss of Independence
- Fatigue
- Nutritional Status
- Stress
- Depression
- Burnout
- Loss of Identity

Finding Joy and Meaning

One way to find joy in the sandwich generation is to focus on the positive aspects of caregiving, such as the opportunity to form close bonds with loved ones and to make a meaningful contribution to their well-being.

Thank you for taking the time to read this book.

Printed in the USA
CPSIA information can be obtained
at www.ICGtesting.com
LVHW012152021024
792708LV00022B/723

9 798330 227297